Naturopathy Diet Plan for Exteme Fat Loss

A Perfect Weight Loss Plan that Works form Breakfast to Dinner, Healthy Eating and Full Day Meal Plan

Dan Phillips PhD

~DEDICATION~

~LARRY~

For your unwavering support, encouragement, and friendship. Your presence in my life has been a constant source of inspiration. Thank you for your invaluable kindness and belief in my journey. This book is a token of appreciation for your enduring friendship and steadfast encouragement.

TABLE OF CONTENT

°°Part I: Introduction to Naturopathy and Extreme Fat Loss°°

1. Introduction to Naturopathy and Extreme Fat Loss
   ° Overview of naturopathy principles and its focus on holistic health
   ° Significance of extreme fat loss and its impact on overall well-being

°°Part II: Understanding the Science of Weight Loss°°

2. Understanding the Science of Weight Loss
   ° How the body stores and burns fat
   ° Metabolism, calorie balance, and the role of hormones in weight loss

7. Crafting a Wholesome Dinner for Optimal Fat Loss

° Guidance on creating a balanced dinner that supports fat loss while ensuring satiety

° Sample dinner recipes emphasizing lean proteins, colorful vegetables, and portion control

°°Part VIII: A Comprehensive Full Day Meal Plan for Extreme Fat Loss°°

8. A Comprehensive Full Day Meal Plan for Extreme Fat Loss

° Detailed meal plan that brings together breakfast, lunch, snacks, and dinner

° Practical tips for adhering to the plan, staying hydrated, and adjusting it to individual needs

CHAPTER 1

Introduction to Naturopathy and Extreme Fat Loss

The quest of health and wellness has become paramount in today's hectic environment. Of all the methods available for attaining the highest possible state of health, naturopathy is unique in that it stresses the body's inherent capacity for self-healing and is comprehensive and holistic. This chapter explores the basic ideas of naturopathy and how it relates to excessive weight loss as well as its significant effects on general health.

Comprehending Naturopathy: A Comprehensive Method for Well-Being

The goal of naturopathy, as a medical philosophy and methodology, is to prevent and promote health by harnessing the healing power of nature. Naturopathy, which dates back to the late 1800s, is a broad field of medicine that uses many techniques to help the body repair itself by promoting its life force. The understanding that the body, mind, and spirit are interrelated and that striking a balance in these areas is crucial to attaining optimal health is one of the fundamental tenets of naturopathy.

Practitioners of naturopathy place a strong emphasis on customized treatment regimens that go beyond masking symptoms to address the underlying causes of health problems. These regimens frequently involve hydrotherapy, herbal medicines, dietary changes, and lifestyle improvements. Naturopathy takes a comprehensive approach to health, aiming to prevent future ailments in addition to treating current ones.

High-Level Fat Loss: Revealing Its Importance

A key component of achieving health and wellbeing is managing weight. Numerous health problems, such as diabetes, joint troubles, and cardiovascular disease, have been connected to excess body fat. Many people aim for fat loss because they understand how important it is to

maintain a healthy weight and how
it can enhance their overall quality
of life.

The main focus of this book is
extreme fat loss, which goes
beyond conventional methods of
weight loss. To become leaner and
healthier, a considerable quantity of
body fat must be lost. Although the
desire for a more attractive
appearance frequently serves as a
driving force, excessive fat
reduction has far more important
implications.

Comprehensive Effects of Severe Fat Loss on General Well-Being

Extreme weight loss and general well-being have a complex relationship. From a physiological standpoint, losing extra weight can result in better insulin sensitivity, less inflammation, and a lower chance of developing chronic illnesses. Cardiovascular health tends to improve with decreasing body fat percentage because it improves blood circulation and lessens the workload on the heart.

Moreover, severe weight reduction may have a negative effect on one's mental and emotional health. Many people who reach their weight loss objectives report feeling more confident and having a better body image. This increased self-assurance frequently has a ripple effect on relationships, professional success, and personal development.

Naturopathy is in perfect harmony with the extreme fat loss tenets when viewed holistically. Naturopathy offers a sustainable and harmonious approach to supporting the quest for extreme fat loss by emphasizing the body's innate capacity for self-healing and self-rebalancing. Naturopathy encourages a progressive, steady approach that takes into account each person's specific needs, challenges, and goals, as opposed to intensive workout regimes or crash diets.

In summary, severe fat reduction is about attaining a state of well-being that includes physical, mental, and emotional harmony. This is in line with naturopathy's emphasis on holistic health. This all-encompassing viewpoint lays the groundwork for a life-changing path towards drastic weight loss that is based on long-term vitality, self-acceptance, and self-care.

We will go into the specifics of naturopathy's function in extreme fat loss in the upcoming chapters. We will explore the naturopathic concepts that underpin our methodology in further detail, as well as the methods and techniques that can support you in achieving significant weight loss while enhancing your general health. Your body, mind, and soul are all interrelated during this journey, which will ultimately result in a healthier, happier, and more vibrant version of yourself.

CHAPTER 2

Understanding the Science of Weight Loss

Studying the complex processes governing our body's use and storage of fat is essential if we are to achieve a healthier lifestyle and a more ideal body weight. The field of weight loss science is broad and involves intricate interactions between hormonal control, metabolic dynamics, and physiological processes. In order to shed light on the mechanisms that propel our bodies to lose excess weight and attain a balanced state of well-being, Chapter 2 of our exploration into this science aims to solve the puzzles surrounding fat storage and metabolism.

Storage and Use of Fat: A Careful Balance

Over thousands of years, our bodies have changed to become more adept at storing and using energy for survival. Fat is one of the main materials the body uses to store energy because it's a concentrated and easily accessible fuel source. Adipose tissue, also known as body fat, is made up of specialized cells called adipocytes that store fat. Our ancestors had to store energy during times of abundance to support them through times of scarcity, so they inherited this survival mechanism—storing fat.

This delicate balance has been upset by the modern environment, which is marked by easy access to high-calorie foods and sedentary lifestyles. Overconsumption of calories and insufficient exercise can tip the balances in favor of body fat buildup, which can result in overweight and obesity.

Metabolism: The Weight-Regulating Engine

The complex web of chemical reactions that our bodies go through to stay alive is called metabolism. It is made up of two primary parts: catabolism, which is the breakdown of molecules to release energy, and anabolism, which is the construction of molecules and storage of energy. Our metabolism is a major factor in determining whether we gain, decrease, or stay the same weight when it comes to weight control.

The amount of energy used by the body at rest to sustain vital processes like breathing, circulation, and cellular activity is known as the basal metabolic rate, or BMR. Age, gender, heredity, and body composition are some of the variables that affect BMR. The total energy expenditure also includes the effects of physical activity and the thermic impact of food (TEF).

Calorie Balance: The Secret to Losing Weight

The basic idea of calorie balance is at the core of weight loss. According to this theory, weight loss happens when energy expenditure is greater than energy intake. To put it another way, when the body needs more calories than it is putting in, it experiences a calorie deficit which forces the body to use its fat reserves as a source of energy and eventually causes weight loss.

Increasing physical activity and making dietary changes together can help create a calorie deficit. Excessively restricted diets or intense exercise routines can cause metabolic adaptations that impede long-term weight loss attempts, therefore a sustainable and balanced strategy is essential.

Hormones: The Harmonious Orchestra of Body Mass Control

Numerous hormones work together in a complicated orchestra to regulate weight; each hormone has a unique effect on hunger, metabolism, and fat accumulation. The pancreas secretes insulin, which is essential for controlling blood sugar levels. It encourages the storage of extra glucose as fat and makes it easier for cells to absorb glucose for energy. Weight gain can be attributed to insulin dysregulation, which is frequently observed in disorders such as insulin resistance.

Fat cells produce leptin, also referred to as the "satiety hormone," which alerts the brain when we are satisfied. However, the "hunger hormone" generated by the stomach that increases appetite is called ghrelin. Our perceptions of hunger and fullness are governed by the intricate interplay of these hormones, which impacts our food preferences and total energy consumption.

The "stress hormone," cortisol, is released in reaction to a variety of stimuli. Although its original function was to release energy in times of fight-or-flight, long-term stress and high cortisol levels can cause an increase in hunger and the storage of fat, especially around the abdomen.

The Intricate Interaction: Applying Science to Practice

Becoming knowledgeable about the science of weight loss involves more than just being aware of physiological processes. It gives people the tools they need to make wise decisions and gives them the confidence to choose sensible plans for reaching and keeping a healthy weight. A holistic strategy for managing weight takes into account the complex interactions between metabolism and hormone control and balances food, exercise, and lifestyle changes.

Finally, Chapter 2 explores the complex network of variables influencing weight loss, providing a thorough analysis of fat storage, metabolism, calorie balance, and the critical function hormones play. Equipped with this insight, people can manage their weight by navigating the path with a deeper comprehension of the systems that support their journey. Chapter 2 gives us the knowledge and skills we need to make wise decisions and start along a sustainable route to a more balanced and healthy lifestyle as we continue our investigation.

CHAPTER 3

Building a Solid Foundation:

Healthy Eating Habits

One cannot stress the importance of developing healthy eating habits in a world full of fad diets and fast fixes. This chapter explores the fundamentals of portion management, mindful eating, and balanced nutrition, highlighting the significance of developing a healthy relationship with food and avoiding emotional eating. A strong foundation of healthful eating practices can help people set themselves up for long-term, successful weight loss and general wellbeing.

Eating with Mindfulness: Its Power

During meals, mindful eating is a technique that is based on awareness, attentiveness, and presence. It's simple to fall into the habit of wolfing down meals quickly in our fast-paced lifestyles, without appreciating or realizing the sustenance they offer. People who practice mindful eating are encouraged to take their time, use all of their senses, and enjoy their meals to the fullest.

People who engage in mindful eating become more aware of their bodies' signals of hunger and fullness. Since they are more likely to know when they are truly full, this awareness helps prevent overeating. dining with awareness also helps one to develop a greater appreciation for the tastes, smells, and textures of food, which makes dining a pleasurable sensory experience.

Combining Control Over Portion

One important but frequently disregarded component of eating healthfully is portion control. It's critical to reclaim control over the amount of food we eat at a time where excessive serving sizes are the standard. Portion control is watching how much food is served and realizing that bigger servings don't always translate into happier customers.

Acquiring the ability to determine suitable serving sizes enables people to efficiently control their caloric consumption. In the context of significant fat loss, this is especially important because portion control can result in a steady and gradual loss of weight. People can establish a calorie deficit while still giving their bodies the vital nutrients they require by combining portion management with a balanced diet.

Well-Balanced Diet for Maximum Health

The foundation of healthy eating practices is balanced nutrition, which is giving the body a wide range of nutrients that it needs to function properly. A varied range of dietary groups, such as lean proteins, complex carbs, healthy fats, and an abundance of vitamins and minerals, are included in a balanced diet.

People can make sure their bodies get the nutrients they need for energy, metabolism, and general health by eating a well-rounded diet. Furthermore, balanced meals help maintain muscle mass during the fat loss process, avoiding the loss of lean mass that is frequently linked to restrictive diets.

Building a Healthful Connection with Food

Maintaining a healthy connection with food is essential for long-term weight loss and general well-being. This entails escaping the vicious cycle of emotional attachment, guilt, and humiliation that can accompany eating behaviors. Food should not be viewed as a source of stress or reward, but rather as nourishment and enjoyment.

Reframing negative eating attitudes, practicing self-compassion, and allowing for occasional indulgences guilt-free are all helpful strategies for creating a happy connection with food. People can lower their risk of binge eating episodes and keep a healthier mindset by eating in a balanced and flexible manner.

Disturbing Emotional Eating

The most well-intentioned attempts to lose weight can be derailed by emotional eating, which is frequently brought on by stress, depression, or boredom. It's critical to distinguish between emotional desires and actual hunger. Developing a social network, finding stress-relieving activities to do, and practicing relaxation techniques are some strategies to prevent emotional eating.

In conclusion, the key to both effective fat loss and overall wellbeing is laying a strong foundation of healthful eating habits. People who practice mindful eating, portion control, balanced nutrition, and have a positive relationship with food are more equipped to make long-lasting decisions that support their weight loss objectives. By adhering to these guidelines, readers can start a life-changing path toward drastic weight loss while fostering a healthy relationship with their bodies and the food they eat.

CHAPTER 4

Designing an Effective Breakfast for Fat Loss

The path to fat loss involves both practical application and an awareness of the underlying science. Creating a meal that sets the tone for the day is an important step in this process. The art and science of creating a nutrient-rich breakfast that boosts metabolism, offers long-lasting energy, and aids in fat loss are covered in detail in Chapter 4. This chapter examines a variety of breakfast options and provides sample dishes in an effort to help readers make decisions that will maximize their mornings and help them reach their weight reduction objectives.

The Boost to Metabolism Through Nutrient-Rich Breakfast Options

The phrase "most important meal of the day" is applied to breakfast for a purpose. It gives the nutrition you need to power your activities and revs up your metabolism after a night of fasting. Dietary choices that are high in nutrients can have a big impact on fat loss. A balanced diet that includes the three macronutrients—fats, proteins, and carbohydrates—can help control blood sugar, reduce appetite, and encourage the burning of fat.

Inspirational Breakfast Recipes: Combining Nutrients to Lose Weight

1. Oliver & Yogurt Plate:

- Greek yogurt, which is high in probiotics and protein.

- Fresh berries, which are high in fiber and antioxidants

Chia seeds: a good source of fiber and healthful fats

- Walnuts or almonds (which add crunch and beneficial fats)

- A honey drizzle (for sweetness from nature)

The vivid flavors of berries and the crunch of almonds are combined with the creamy texture of Greek yogurt in this parfait. The fiber aids in digestion and keeps you feeling full, and the protein from the yogurt and the good fats from the nuts and chia seeds help you feel full.

2. Egg Toast and Avocado: - Whole-grain or sprouted-grain bread (high in fiber and complex carbs)

- Avocado: monounsaturated fats can be found there.

- Scrambled or poached eggs (excellent source of protein)

- Kale or spinach (with extra minerals and vitamins)

This delicious choice combines the protein-dense eggs with the creamy avocado. Leafy greens add an extra nutritional boost while whole-grain bread sustains energy. Nutritious fats and protein work together to keep you full all morning long.

3. Banana and Nut Butter Oatmeal:

Rolled oats (high in fiber and complex carbs)

- Nut butter, for protein and healthy fats (try almond or peanut butter).

- Banana slices (natural potassium and sweetness)

- Cinnamon (which enhances flavor and could help control blood sugar)

A basic breakfast option, oatmeal is made even better with the addition of banana slices and nut butter. Protein, healthy fats, and carbs work together to create a balanced meal that boosts energy and reduces cravings.

4. Smoothie Bowl: - Frozen mixed berries rich in fiber and antioxidants

- Kale or spinach (for minerals and vitamins)

– Protein powder (to add even more protein to meals)

- Almond milk without sugar (for hydration and a creamy base)

- Almond slices, coconut flakes, and chia seeds as garnishes

A customized and refreshing alternative is a smoothie bowl. A foundation rich in nutrients is created by adding protein powder, mixed berries, and leafy greens. Additions such as sliced almonds and chia seeds enhance the dish's texture and nutritional value.

Achieving Success through Harmonizing Taste and Nutrition

Finding the right mix between nutrients and taste is key to creating a meal that helps people lose weight. To accommodate a range of tastes and dietary requirements, these sample breakfast recipes include a diversity of flavors, textures, and nutrients. A combination of fiber-rich foods, lean proteins, healthy fats, and complex carbohydrates sets the stage for a day of thoughtful eating and sustained energy in these breakfast alternatives.

Chapter Four provides readers with useful tools to help them make educated breakfast choices as they go out on their fat loss quest. Through the selection of nutrient-dense foods that enhance metabolism, facilitate fullness, and encourage fat reduction, people can develop a healthy and enduring weight-management strategy. With the help of these delectable and filling breakfast recipes, readers will feel more equipped to welcome mornings as a chance to fuel their activities, energize their bodies, and advance their desired fat loss goals.

CHAPTER 5

Lunchtime Choices for Sustained Energy and Fat Burning

Lunch is a critical time to replenish bodily energy and maintain a high level of energy all day. The techniques for creating midday meals that both avoid energy crashes and speed up the burning of fat are covered in this chapter.

Lunch meals that include plant-based protein sources, high-fiber veggies, and healthy fats help people maximize their nutrition and make progress toward their severe weight loss objectives.

Maintaining Vitality with Well-Selected Lunch Items

A regular occurrence is the midday slump, which is frequently linked to unbalanced meals that alter blood sugar levels. Selecting a meal that will keep the metabolism going and giving you prolonged energy is crucial to preventing this energy slump. This is especially important for people who are trying to lose a lot of weight because steady energy levels encourage regular exercise and healthy metabolism.

Power of Plant-Based Proteins

A meal must include protein, but it's especially important around noon. There are several advantages to include plant-based protein sources including lentils, quinoa, tofu, and tempeh. In comparison to certain animal-based proteins, plant-based proteins are lower in saturated fats and higher in essential amino acids.

Eating a sufficient amount of protein at lunchtime ensures that the body uses stored fat as its primary source of energy and preserves lean muscle mass during the fat loss process. Furthermore, consuming foods high in protein makes you feel fuller for longer, which lowers the chance of overindulging later in the day.

High-Fiber Vegetables to Aid in Satiety

A useful tool in the fight against overindulgence and weight gain is fiber. Broccoli, spinach, kale, and bell peppers are examples of high-fiber veggies that give meals body without adding extra calories. They help create sensations of fullness and contentment, which reduces the likelihood of consuming additional calories later in the day.

Additionally, fiber is essential for healthy digestion and gut flora, which promotes general wellbeing. When people include a range of vibrant veggies in their lunch meals, they boost their nutritional intake and aid in weight loss by decreasing caloric intake and improving digestion.

Unleashing the Potential of Good Fats

In the context of fat loss, the word "fat" may sound contradictory, but good fats are necessary for both weight management and optimal health. Meals are more satiating and flavorful when sources of healthy fats like avocados, nuts, seeds, and olive oil are included in the lunchtime recipes.

In addition to being high in calories, healthy fats improve the body's absorption of nutrients and help the body use vitamins and minerals. Additionally, they help to maintain constant blood sugar levels, which averts energy dumps that can impair motivation and productivity.

Inspirational Lunch Recipes for Dramatic Fat Loss

1. Asparagus and Quinoa Salad: A zesty concoction of cooked quinoa, cucumbers, tomatoes, red onions, olives, and feta cheese, topped with

a lemon-olive oil drizzle. This dish provides a range of nutrients, plant-based protein, and healthy fats.

2. Stir-fried Tofu and Veggies: Stir-fry with colorful bell peppers, broccoli, snap peas, and tofu cubes sautéed in a tasty sauce prepared with ginger, garlic, and low-sodium soy sauce. For extra fiber, serve over a bed of brown rice.

3. Avocado and Chickpea Wrap: A whole wheat wrap topped with shredded carrots, spinach, avocado slices, mashed chickpeas, and pumpkin seeds. For lunch on-the-

go, this protein-rich wrap is a quick and filling choice.

Including these lunchtime options in a fat reduction strategy helps to enhance metabolism, encourage prolonged energy, and increase feelings of fullness all day long. Plant-based proteins, high-fiber veggies, and healthy fats are the main ways that people can improve their nutrition and eat in a way that supports their overall health and extreme weight loss objectives.

CHAPTER 6

Snacking Smart: Nutrient-Packed Options for Extreme Fat Loss

Every element of a person's food decisions is vital in the quest for extreme fat loss. Of these, snacking stands out as a crucial element that has the power to either facilitate or obstruct achievement. The importance of snacking for regulating blood sugar, reducing cravings, and supplying long-lasting energy is covered in detail in Chapter 6. This chapter attempts to assist readers in making wise decisions that will help them on their path to dramatic weight loss by providing a thorough list of nutrient-dense snack ideas.

Snacking's Function in Maintaining Steady Blood Sugar Levels

Not only does snacking help to bridge the time between meals, but it also helps to keep blood sugar levels steady. An increase in appetite, energy dumps, and overeating might result from blood sugar levels that swing dramatically as a result of irregular eating schedules or sugary snack use. Nutrient-dense, well-planned snacks, particularly high in fiber and protein, help control blood sugar levels and avoid these unfavorable peaks and valleys.

Healthy Snack Ideas for Dramatic Fat Loss

1. Hummus and Veggie Sticks: - Hummus is a good source of healthy fats and protein.

   - Sticks of bell pepper, cucumber, and carrot (fiber and vitamins)

2. Hard-Boiled Eggs: - Poached eggs with a high protein content and beneficial fats

3. Probiotic-rich Greek Yogurt with Berries: - Greek yogurt

   - Fresh berries (high in fiber and antioxidants)

4. Edamame: - Gently cooked edamame (a plant-based source of fiber and protein).

5. Walnuts or Almonds: - Uncooked walnuts or almonds (satisfying crunch and healthful fats)

6. Nutty Butter on Apple Slices:

   - Sliced apples (naturally sweet and high in fiber)

   - Nut butter (protein and good fats)

7. Fruit and Cottage Cheese: - Fruit (protein)

  - Sliced berries or peaches (for taste and fiber)

8. Fried Rice Cakes with Avocado: - Fried rice cakes with a crispy, low-calorie foundation

  - Slices of avocado (good fats)

9. Trail Mix: - A combination of dried fruit, nuts, and seeds that is filling and high in energy.

10. Mini Wrap with Cheese and Veggies:

- Wholegrain mini wrap with fiber and complex carbs

- Cubed cheese (taste and protein)

- Cucumber, tomato, and lettuce slices (for nutrients and fiber)

Enhancing Weight Loss With Informed Snacking

A comprehensive approach is necessary for the trip toward extreme fat loss, and wise snacking is a useful tool within this framework. This chapter's selection of nutrient-dense snack ideas offers a wide range of tastes, textures, and nutrients to suit a variety of dietary requirements and preferences. These snacks are made with a blend of fiber-rich, protein-rich, and healthy fats to help control blood sugar, increase fullness, and prevent cravings.

People who are starting on the path of extreme fat reduction can improve their overall progress, energy levels, and metabolism by choosing their snacks wisely. Making sensible snacking decisions that fuel the body, assist fat reduction objectives, and promote a long-term weight management strategy is what smart snacking is all about—not deprivation. Chapter 6 equips readers to embrace eating as a strategic weapon in their goal of extreme fat loss as they peruse the variety of nutrient-dense snack alternatives, ultimately encouraging a sense of control, contentment, and achievement on their transforming journey.

CHAPTER 7

Crafting a Wholesome Dinner for Optimal Fat Loss

- Guidance on creating a balanced dinner that supports fat loss while ensuring satiety.

- Sample dinner recipes emphasizing lean proteins, colorful vegetables, and portion control.

Dinner is a vital chance to fuel the body and support satiety and fat reduction as the day comes to an end. This chapter explores the skill of preparing dinners that are both balanced and supportive of significant weight loss. Through the use of lean meats, colorful veggies, and portion restriction, people may make sure that their evening meal supports their overall health and weight loss goals.

Tips for a Well-Rounded Dinner

Since dinner is the last major meal before a time of fasting during sleep, it has a special role in the fat loss path. Creating a well-balanced meal not only helps supply vital nutrients but also promotes a sound sleep, which is important for metabolism and general health.

Lean Proteins to Preserve Muscle

A supper meal focused on weight loss must include lean protein sources like turkey, fish, or grilled chicken, as well as plant-based options like tofu and beans. Foods high in protein aid in the development and repair of lean muscle mass, avoiding muscle mass loss during the weight reduction process. Sustaining muscle mass is essential since it raises the body's resting metabolic rate and improves its capacity for burning calories.

Vegetables with Color to Boost Nutrient Density

Vegetables with vibrant colors are not only eye-catching but also nutrient- and mineral-rich. Including a range of veggies in supper recipes guarantees a nutrient-dense diet that promotes both weight control and general wellness.

Try to include a variety of hues on your dish, such as brightly colored peppers, dark greens, carrots, and broccoli. Fiber from these veggies promotes fullness and helps with digestion, both of which help with portion control.

Portion Control: An Important Elements

Controlling portion sizes is especially important during supper because eating too much in the evening can cause digestive problems and poor sleep. It's critical to pay attention to portion sizes and learn to distinguish between fullness and satisfaction.

Using smaller bowls or plates can assist provide the impression of a bigger plate without adding too many calories. This is one useful tactic. Furthermore, give yourself time to eat carefully, enjoy every meal, and listen to your body's cues about when it is suitably full.

Recipe Examples for Losing Weight at Dinner

1. Steamed vegetables and quinoa with grilled salmon: A salmon fillet that is cooked to perfection and presented with quinoa on the side and a mixture of steamed broccoli, carrots, and asparagus. This recipe provides a good ratio of complex carbohydrates, lean protein, and nutrient-dense veggies.

2. Stir-fried Vegetables with Lentils: A plant-based stir-fry with mixed vegetables, cooked lentils, and a tasty sauce made with low-sodium soy sauce, ginger, and garlic. Serve this delightful low-

carb choice over a bed of cauliflower rice.

3. Stuffed Bell Peppers: Vibrant bell peppers stuffed with quinoa, diced tomatoes, black beans, lean ground turkey, and seasonings. This meal, when baked to perfection and garnished with a dollop of low-fat cheese, is savory and filling.

Making these healthful meal selections helps the body receive the vital nutrients it needs to achieve fat loss goals. Lean proteins, vibrant veggies, and portion control are priorities that can help people make the best meal choices for their overall health and successful journey toward extreme fat loss.

CHAPTER 8

A Comprehensive Full Day Meal Plan for Extreme Fat Loss

- A detailed meal plan that brings together breakfast, lunch, snacks, and dinner.

- Practical tips for adhering to the plan, staying hydrated, and adjusting it to individual needs.

Starting an intensive fat reduction journey necessitates a planned and well-rounded nutritional strategy. This chapter includes a full-day meal plan that will help you reach your weight loss objectives by integrating breakfast, lunch, snacks, and dinner in a smooth manner. In addition to providing nutrition, this carefully thought-out meal plan also helps regulate blood sugar, reduce cravings, and maximize energy for your quest for dramatic weight loss. With helpful advice on sticking to the diet, staying hydrated, and personalizing it, this meal plan is an invaluable road map that will lead you to success.

Sunday Breakfast: Berry Yogurt Parfait

Greek yogurt: a source of probiotics and protein

- Berries that are mixed (fiber and antioxidants)

– Chia seeds (rich in fiber and good fats)

- A drizzle of honey for sweetness naturally

Grilled Chicken Salad for Lunch

- Lean protein grilled chicken breast

- Mixed greens with vitamins and fiber

Tomato, bell pepper, and cucumber (added nutrients)

- A dressing of olive oil and vinegar (healthy fats)

Afternoon Snack: Apple Slices with Nut Butter

- Sliced apples (naturally sweet and high in fiber)

- Nut butter (protein and good fats)

Supper: Quinoa and Vegetable Baked Salmon

- Baked salmon fillet (high in protein and omega-3 fatty acids)
Quinoa (high in protein and complex carbs)
- Steamed carrots and broccoli (rich in fiber and minerals)
Herbs with lemon juice (flavor)

Afternoon snack: Hummus-topped vegetable sticks

- Sticks of carrot, celery, and bell pepper (high in vitamins and fiber)
- Hummus (a healthy fat and protein blend)

Adherence and Customization: Useful Tips

1. Control of Portion: Although the meal plan offers a structure, it is crucial to manage portions. To control your calorie intake, pay attention to portion sizes.

2. Hydration: Throughout the day, sip on lots of water. Maintaining hydration aids with appetite control and metabolism.

3. Pay Attention to Your Body: Observe your body's signals of hunger and fullness. Adapt snack frequency or portion sizes to your body's requirements.

4. Introduction: Tailor the meal plan to your dietary requirements and personal tastes. Change meals or ingredients without altering the nutritional balance overall.

5. Meal Prep: Arrange meals or ingredients ahead of time to guarantee you have wholesome options close at hand and lessen the temptation to choose unhealthy selections.

6. Consistency: To maintain a sustainable approach, adhere to the

meal plan regularly while leaving room for occasional indulgences.

7. Mindful Eating: To increase satisfaction, practice mindful eating by slowing down, enjoying every bite, and being present when you eat.

8. Physical Activity: To maximize fat loss and general well-being, combine your diet plan with frequent physical activity.

Final Thoughts: Your Plan for Dramatic Fat Loss

This complete meal plan integrates nutrient-dense meals into each meal and snack to help your journey toward extreme fat loss. It acts as a thorough road map for weight loss. This strategy combines complex carbohydrates, fiber, healthy fats, and protein to maximize energy, stabilize blood sugar, and reduce cravings.

As you go out on this journey of transformation, never forget that adaptability and constancy are your friends. Make use of the helpful advice given to customize the menu to your own requirements and tastes. You may take control of your fat loss journey and work towards reaching your chosen objectives by following this meal plan, drinking enough of water, and engaging in mindful eating.

In the end, Chapter 8 acts as a compass, pointing you in the direction of a sustainable, well-balanced strategy to severe fat reduction while encouraging a sense of accomplishment, empowerment, and control as you travel the road to a healthier and more energetic version of yourself.

www.ingramcontent.com/pod-product-compliance
Lightning Source LLC
Chambersburg PA
CBHW060751260726
48660CB00002B/576